# KETO DIET FOR BEGINNER'S

Guide to Low Carb Recipes for Weight Loss
and 21 Day Meal Plan

JENNIFER AXE

# Keto Diet for Beginners

*Guide to Low Carb Recipes for Weight Loss*
*And*
*21-Day Meal Plan*

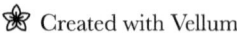 Created with Vellum

## Introduction

Thank you for grabbing a copy of *Keto for Beginners*.

The Ketogenic Diet derives from the metabolic process known as *ketosis,* which forces your body to use fat as fuel. This diet uses fat as a quicker and easier way to shed unwanted pounds by reducing your intake of carbs and excess sugars.

The following chapters will discuss some of the many reasons why you should make the choice to feel better about yourself, both inside and out, *today*, through the means of this successful diet!

You will discover how important it is to balance out your carb intake so that your body will have more room for foods higher in fat that our bodies can use as a better source of fuel. If you have not been previously privy to what the ketogenic diet has to offer, you are in for a real treat!

This diet is not a fad or a trend; it is one of the most utilized diets on the market! Your success solely depends on your willpower to steer clear from foods that do not provide your body with the proper fuel to be the best you can be.

Within this book lie the basics of the ketogenic diet so you can wrap your mind around the grand concepts. You're still not sure where to start? No worries! This book is packed with a plethora of recipes to get you started on the right foot!

There are plenty of books about the ketogenic diet on the market, so thanks again for choosing this one! Every effort was made to ensure it is full of as much useful information as possible. What are you waiting for? Dive in and start the process of becoming a healthier version of yourself! Good luck!

# How the Ketogenic Diet Works

If you have purchased this book with not one clue as to what the Ketogenic Diet is, do not fret! This chapter will discuss and go into some detail about the most crucial aspects as to what makes this diet so successful!

## What is the Ketogenic Diet?

The phrase 'ketogenic' is stemmed from the natural process of 'ketosis', which allows our bodies to thrive when the intake of food might be low. Ketones are produced during this process as fats in our livers break down. The entire goal of the ketogenic diet is to force our bodies to stay within this state of high metabolism.

No, it is not about starving yourself and keeping yourself from consuming food, but rather the starvation of consuming carbohydrates. Humans have not changed in the fact that we can adapt to our environments at drastic speeds. When you pack your body with bad edibles, it will start to burn those precious ketones that are partially responsible for weight loss and optimum mental and physical performance.

## The Birth of the Keto Diet

The ketogenic diet has been around for quite a few decades. It was developed by a guy named Dr. Russell Wilder back in the year 1924. It was quite the concoction that treated epilepsy but unfortunately fell through due to the creation of anti-seizure medications that came about during the 1940s. It didn't make much of an appearance until the mid-1990, when the Abraham family began the Charlie Foundation for their son, Charlie. Charlie's body did not handle that entire anti-seizure pill-popping very well. He began following the means of the ketogenic diet as a toddler and stuck to it for a time period of five years. He is now a successful college student and is still, to this day, seizure-free.

The bottom line is that the ketogenic diet is made up of extremely low-carb and high-fat intakes. This diet is quite like that of the Atkins and other low-carb diets. While you are reducing your intake of carbohydrates by such drastic amounts, you are replacing it with foods high in fat.

The absence of carbs creates a higher metabolic state within your body, known as ketosis (as mentioned above.) In Layman's terms, our body becomes an incredibly powered working machine, burning off fat for energy instead of ketones. It warps our metabolisms so that it no longer burns precious substances utilized to keep our bodies in the best shape they can be.

This diet has been shown to reduce blood sugars and insulin levels which make it a diet that is loaded with quite a few health benefits. You will read about some of these benefits later in this chapter.

## Different Types of Ketogenic Diets

- **High-protein ketogenic diet** – This form of the

keto-diet is the same but involved consuming more protein. The ratio required to stick to this diet is 60% fat, 35% protein, and 5% carbohydrates.

- **Targeted ketogenic diet (TKD)** – This diet allows wiggle room to consume a bit more carbs if they revolve around workouts.
- **Cyclical ketogenic diet (CKD)** – This form of the keto-diet requires periods of high-carb intakes, such as 5 ketogenic days followed by a couple of high-carb intake days.
- **Standard ketogenic diet (SKD)** – This diet is the most utilized and recommended and requires one to consume moderate amounts of protein and high-fat. It usually involves 75% fat, 20% protein, and 5% carbs.

The standard ketogenic version of the diet is the most sought out and recommended, as well as the most researched. The others are usually utilized by advanced individuals, such as athletes and bodybuilders.

## Foods You Can Eat on the Ketogenic Diet

- Grass-fed and wild animal sources:
- Beef
- Lamb
- Goat
- Venison
- Fish and seafood
- Pork
- Poultry
- Eggs
- Gelatin

- Ghee
- Liver, heart, kidneys, and other organ meats
- Healthy fats:
- Saturated
- Coconut oil
- Butter
- Ghee
- Goose fat
- Duck fat
- Chicken fat
- Tallow
- Lard
- Monounsaturated
- Olive oil
- Macadamia oil
- Avocado oil
- Polyunsaturated
- Fatty fish and seafood
- Non-starchy veggies
- Leafy greens
- Radicchio
- Endive
- Chives
- Chard
- Lettuce
- Spinach
- Bok choy
- Swiss chard
- Cruciferous vegetables
- Radishes
- Kohlrabi
- Dark leaf kale
- Celery

- Asparagus
- Cucumber
- Summer squash (spaghetti squash, zucchini)
- Bamboo shoots
- Fruits:
- Avocado
- Beverages and Condiments:
- Water
- Black coffee
- Tea
- Pork rinds
- Mayo
- Mustard
- Pesto
- Bone broth
- Pickles and other fermented eats
- Spices
- Lemon/lime juice & zest
- Whey protein

## Eat on Occasion

- Vegetables and fruits:
- Berries (mulberries, cranberries, raspberries, strawberries, blueberries, blackberries, etc.)
- Sugar snap peas
- Artichokes
- Water chestnuts
- Sea vegetables
- Root veggies (pumpkin, winter squash, mushrooms, etc.)
- Cabbage
- Cauliflower

- Broccoli
- Fennel
- Brussels sprouts
- Full-fat dairy
- Nuts and seeds:
- Sunflower seeds
- Pecans, almonds, walnuts, hazelnuts, etc.
- Macadamia nuts

## Foods to Avoid on the Keto Diet

- Grains
- Rice, corn, oats, wheat, barley, etc.
- Pasta, breads, cookies, crackers, etc.
- Factory-farmed fish and pork
- Processed foods
- Artificial sweeteners
- Refined fats and oils
- Foods that are "low-fat", "low-carb" or "zero-carb"
- Milk
- Alcoholic and sweet beverages
- Tropical fruits and fruit juices
- Soy products

## Understanding Fats on the Ketogenic

Since fats make up over 70% of the daily macros you are to consume on the ketogenic diet, they are vital to your success while on this diet. But it is not just consuming fat that this is crucial, but choosing the right fats is important as well! There can be a lot of confusion as to what fats are good, bad, and need to be avoided. This chapter will break down the good and bad fats on the keto-genic diet.

## Good Ketogenic Fats

The "good guy" fats that are a go when it comes to the ketogenic diet are split up into 4 different categories:

1. Trans fats
2. Polyunsaturated fats (PUFAs)
3. Monounsaturated fats (MUFAs)
4. Saturated fats

When it boils down to "what types of aspects are in what fats" you must remember that all fats in the world are created by a mixture of all the above types of fat but are categorized by which one is the most dominant. Here, we will break down each type of fat when it comes to consuming foods on the keto diet. This will help you to easily see them when you are making decisions about what to fuel your body and mind with.

## Healthy Saturated Fats

Saturated fats had a bad reputation for many years. They were viewed as terrible for the health of your heart and we were taught to either avoid them or to decrease our consumption of them.

However, since then, there have been various studies to prove this wrong and have shown no significant link between saturated fats to the risk of heart disease. We have been consuming saturated fats for *thousands* of years. In light of this new information, there are a plethora of great benefits that come along with the inclusion of healthy saturated fats in your daily diet.

Many kinds of saturated fat include something we call "medium-chain triglycerides (MCTs)," which coconut oil, small amounts of butter, and palm oil have in them. MCT is easily digestible, for when we eat these MCT's, they pass through the liver and are utilized automatically as an energy source! This means that they are superb things to have in your diet if you want to lose weight or boost your physical performance.

- Health benefits of saturated fats:
- Increase in the function of the immune system
- Better cholesterol levels, both HDL and LDL
- Better HDL to LDL cholesterol ratio
- Improved maintenance of bone density
- A rise of good cholesterol (HDL) to prevent the buildup of LDL
- Promotes the creation of hormones like cortisol and testosterone, which are important for various reasons
- Best sources of saturated fats to eat on the keto:
- Butter
- Cocoa butter
- Coconut oil
- Red meat
- Palm oil
- Lard
- Eggs
- Cream

## Healthy Keto Monounsaturated Fats

MUFAs or monounsaturated fatty acids have been accepted as "good fat" for a long time. There have been a variety of studies that have directly linked MUFAs with benefits such as insulin resistance and good cholesterol levels.

## Health benefits of MUFAs:

- Better levels of HDL cholesterol

- Decrease in blood pressure
- Decreased risk of developing heart disease
- Decrease in belly fat
- Decrease in insulin resistance

## Best sources of MUFAs to eat on the keto:

- Avocados and avocado oil
- Extra virgin olive oil
- Goose fat
- Lard and bacon fat
- Macadamia nut oil

## Healthy Polyunsaturated Fats

When it comes to consuming polyunsaturated fatty acids (PUFAs), it boils most importantly down to the type. When PUFAs are heated up, they can create free radicals, which are harmful to the body and responsible for the increase of inflammation and have been shown to raise the risk of having diseases like cancer. Most PUFAs should be eaten in forms that are cold forms and you should avoid using them for cooking purposes.

PUFAS CAN BE FOUND in processed oils and other extremely healthy sources. Eating the correct kinds of PUFAs can give you benefits, especially when you incorporate them with the ketogenic diet. They include Omega 6's and Omega 3's, which are essential to feeling great!

THE AMOUNT of PUFAs that you eat is extremely crucial. Most

western diets have a PUFA ratio of 1:30, even though the recommended ratio is just 1:1.

## Health benefits of PUFAs:

When you consume a good balance of omega 3 and omega 6, you greatly reduce the risk of developing the following:

- Autoimmune and inflammatory diseases
- Heart disease
- Helps to improve symptoms of depression
- Improves symptoms of ADHD
- Stroke

## Best sources of PUFAs to eat on the keto:

- Avocado oil
- Chia seeds
- Extra virgin olive oil
- Fatty fish and fish oil
- Flaxseeds and flaxseed oil
- Nut oils
- Sesame oil
- Walnuts

## Natural Trans Fats

You are probably questioning the author's intelligence seeing trans fats under the "good" fats category. But it does have a right to be in this section! Yes, the majority of trans fats are wildly unhealthy and can be very harmful to the human body. *Vaccenic acid* is a type of trans fat that is good for you! It is naturally found in foods like dairy products and grass-fed meats.

Vaccenic acid has health benefits including:

- Decrease in the risk of developing diabetes and obesity
- Decreased risk of developing heart disease
- Protection against developing cancer

Best sources of healthy and natural trans fats to eat on the keto:

- Dairy fats such as butter and yogurt
- Grass-fed animal products

## Bad Ketogenic Fats

One of the positive aspects that attract many people to undergo the ketogenic diet is that they can consume lots of satisfying foods and healthy fats. But, lurking around the corner, there are also bad fats that you must keep an eye out for. You want to get rid of and eliminate these pesky guys, so you don't damage your bodily health. One of the key things to remember on the keto diet is that the genuine quality of the food you eat can mean a world of difference when it comes to your diet results.

## Polyunsaturated Fats and Processed Trans Fats

Processed trans fats are a common type of fat that many of you are familiar with. They have the capability of being wildly detrimental to your overall physical well-being.

ARTIFICIAL TRANS FATS are created during the production of food, which occurs when polyunsaturated fats are processed. Choosing PUFAs that are not altered, overheated, unprocessed, or in any such way is important. The processing of PUFAs creates free radicals that are harmful when consumed and they are made from oils that have seeds that are genetically modified.

### Risks of trans fats consumption:

- Bad for gut health
- Increase of bad LDL cholesterol and decrease in the good HDL cholesterol
- Increased risk of developing cancer
- Increased risk of developing heart disease
- Lead cause of inflammatory health issues

### Examples of trans fats to eliminate:

- Hydrogenated oils that are in products like fast food, margarine, crackers, and cookies
- Processed vegetable oils like canola oils, soybean, safflower, sunflower, and cottonseed

## THINGS TO REMEMBER...

Don't fear saturated fats, but instead, opt for fats that are unprocessed. If you avoid oils and fats found in packaged, processed foods that were factory-made, you will be golden and stay on the right track to healthy success on the ketogenic.

KEEP in mind that the entire goal of this diet is to have much better health including not only maintaining the right carb, protein, fat ratio but picking out sources of food that promote your well-being and overall physical health!

## 2

# Keto Diet Benefits and Risks

All types of low-carb diets have been on the table of controversy for quite a few years. It has been said that diets high in fat content would raise cholesterol levels through the roof, causing heart disease, and other bad body ailments. But research has been changing the face of low-carb dieting. It has been shown that amongst other diets, those low-carb ones are the ones that seem to win the race. They are not only a great substitute when trying to lose weight, but they even have other great health benefits, even reducing cholesterol levels. Here are some ways that the Ketogenic Diet could produce some good things in your life!

## Benefits of the Keto Diet

As you have learned, the basis of ketogenic dieting is centered on a diet that is low in the consumption of carbohydrates, low enough to switch your body from using glucose as energy to utilizing fat, which creates ketones that help you to maximize your health and fitness benefits.

In this chapter, you will learn about the vast array of benefits that come along with jumping on the ketogenic train that can help you to feel like a brand new, healthier human being!

### *Suppresses hunger and cravings*

Many diets out there require you to eat less than your body is used to. This means that never-ending hunger pains are bound to strike and at the worst times. This is the main reason people tend to feel miserable while on any diet plan. Diets that are low in carb intake are great because it automatically reduces your appetite. Those who cut carbs and consume more proteins and fat actually eat *fewer* calories.

### *Better potential for losing weight*

It doesn't take a scientist to know that reducing the number of carbs you eat will contribute to weight loss. People who stick within the means of low-carb diets lose weight at a much faster rate than those who are within the means of a low-carb diet. Diets low in carbohydrates tend to help in the reduction of excess water in our bodies, which can add on the pounds. The ketogenic diet reduces insulin levels too, meaning the kidneys are shedding all that excess sodium that can lead to retaining extra weight.

### *Better focused brain*

Ketogenic diets were noted clear back in the 1920s to treat epileptic children. The precise mechanism that aided in seizure prevention still remains a mystery, but many researchers have no doubt that it has to do with the increase of stable neurons in the brain and the increased regulation of the mitochondria and enzymes that make up our brains.

Direct effects of the ketogenic diet when it comes to our mind are:

- Better mental clarity
- Better focus
- Fewer occurrences and intenseness of migraines

### *Ability to fight cancer*

The supplementation of ketones lessens the viability of tumor growth and lengthens the survival of those with metastatic cancer, as well as other cancers, which are currently being researched.

### Prevents heart disease

When you keep your blood glucose levels low and stabilized, the better your entire body! The ketogenic diet helps to prevent high blood pressures and lowers triglyceride levels.

Many see the keto diet as counterintuitive when it comes to erasing the development of heart disease due to the major increase of fat, but it has been found that the consumption of excess carbs, especially fructose, is a key contributor to a high triglyceride level.

### Decreases inflammation

The ketogenic diet is making giant strides in studies that are related to the negative results of inflammation in the body. It has been found to be highly anti-inflammatory and helps with a wide variety of health issues.

Thus, the keto diet helps to treat:

- Arthritis
- Eczema
- Psoriasis
- IBS
- Acne
- Pain
- And more

### Improved energy levels and quality of sleep

Many beginners who undergo the ketogenic diet report that just after a few days that they have a positive increase in energy levels paired with a lack of cravings for carbs and bad fats. This is because the keto stabilizes insulin levels as well as produces a more readily available energy source that our brains and bodily tissues like better.

Improvement of sleep is still a bit of a mystery, however. The ketogenic diet has been proved to improve sleep thanks to the decrease in REM and increasing the slow-wave sleep patterns that are necessary for quality sleep. Researchers believe that the correlation is related to the biochemical shift that occurs in the brain after ketones are used for energy while other bodily tissues are busy burning fats.

### Keep uric acid levels in check

If you have ever experienced kidney stones or gout, then perhaps the ketogenic diet is for you so you never have to deal with these terrible pains again! What causes these painful ailments is the increase in phosphorus, uric acid, and calcium levels in the body. This occurs thanks to not so great genetics, but mainly due to high consumptions of sugar, being overweight, being dehydrated, and eating and drinking items with alcohol and purines, such as meats and beers.

The ketogenic diet works by temporarily allowing uric acid levels to rise, especially during times of dehydration, and then come down over a period of time.

### Better gastrointestinal and gallbladder health

Foods that are grain-based and/or sugary, such as nightshade veggies tend to increase your likelihood of getting heartburn and acid reflux. When you get yourself on a low carb diet, you will find that these ailments drastically improve and may even completely disappear. This is because low carb diets help to eradicate inflammation and autoimmune responses.

### Assisting in women's health

Over the last decade, there has been much research to show that the ketogenic diet plays a vital role in the enhancement of fertility in women. Low carb diets eliminate symptoms such as prolonged or infrequent periods, obesity, and acne.

This is because women are better able to keep their blood sugars stabilized, which results in lower insulin levels throughout the body, allowing hormones to become stable.

### Better eye health

All diabetics will inform you that their disease is detrimental to their eyesight and leads to an increase in the development of cataracts. When you keep your blood sugars low and stable, you will undoubtfully improve your eyesight over time.

### *Improvement in muscle gain and endurance*

Low carb diets, especially the ketogenic, have been shown to promote the gain of muscle, which is why it is a go-to diet for body-builders. It allows people to gain more muscle and lose more fat.

### *Spares losing muscle while curbing metabolic syndrome, obesity, and diabetes*

I am sure you have seen a number of articles that include "diabetes", "ketogenic", and "ketosis" in the title. Ketogenic dieting is very helpful for those with either type 1 or type 2 diabetes for all the reasons that have been previously talked about in this chapter.

- **Therapy for some brain disorders** – There are certain areas of our brains that strictly run on glucose as a fuel. This is the reason behind why our livers produce it from protein if we do not consume carbs. There are bigger portions of our brains, however, that burn through ketones. Think back to Charlie Abraham, who was mentioned earlier in this chapter. In studies, more than half of children who utilized the ketogenic diet had a 50% reduction in seizures. This diet, among other low-carb diets, is being studied as to what its effect is on brain disorders like Parkinson's and Alzheimer's disease.

## Risks of the Keto Diet

Just like with every good thing in the world, there are some risk factors to consider before diving head first on your journey with the ketogenic diet.

### *Fatigue and irritability*

Even though raised ketone levels can drastically improve a few areas regarding your physical quality of life, they are also directly related to feeling tired and having to work harder during physical activities.

### "Brain Fog"

If you stay on the ketogenic diet long term, there is going to be some major shifting when it comes to the metabolic areas of the body. This can make you moody and somewhat sluggish, which can make you not able to think clearly or adequately focus. Ensure that you are reducing your levels of carb intake at steady levels, not all at once.

### Lipids may fluctuate

Even though fats on the ketogenic diet are welcomed, if you consume large amounts of saturated fats, your cholesterol levels will begin to increase. Make sure you are consuming healthy fats.

### Micronutrient deficiencies

Diets that consist of low-carb foods are more than likely lacking in essential nutrients, such as magnesium, potassium, and iron. You might want to strongly consider finding a high-quality multivitamin to take daily.

### Development of ketoacidosis

If your ketone levels become too wacky, it may lead to this condition. pH levels within your blood decrease, creating an environment that is high in acidity, which can be threatening for those with diabetes.

### Muscle loss

As you consume less energy, your body leans on the help of other tissues as a source of fuel. When working out heavily while on a diet like the ketogenic, there is the potential for major muscle loss.

# 3

# Ultimate Keto Diet Shopping List

## Ketogenic Vegetables

Artichokes
Cucumbers
Asparagus
Eggplant
Avocados
Spinach
Bean Sprouts
Green bell peppers
Bell peppers (Any color)
Green onions
Bok Choy
Greens
Broccoli
Hot peppers
Romaine lettuce
Iceberg lettuce
Cabbage

Leeks
Artichoke hearts
Mushrooms
Asparagus
Napa cabbage
Spaghetti squash
Okra
Spinach
Portabella mushrooms
Green olives
Radishes
Collard greens
Brussel Sprouts
Mushrooms
Snow peas
Pickles
Black olives
Sauerkraut
Green beans
Cauliflower
Zucchini
Celery
Yellow onions

## Ketogenic Fruits

Apples
Mango
Apricot
Melons
Avocados
Nectarines
Bananas
Olives

Blackberries
Oranges
Blueberries
Papaya
Cherries
Passionfruit
Fresh cranberries
Peaches
Dates
Pears
Figs
Pineapple
Grapefruit
Plums
Guava
Pomegranates
Kiwi
Raspberries
Lemons
Rhubarb
Limes
Strawberries
Tangerines
Tomatoes (all types)

## Ketogenic Dairy

Cheddar cheese
Colby cheese
Brie cheese
Cottage cheese
Blue cheese
Feta cheese
Full-fat/full cream milk

Goat cheese
Full-fat/full cream Greek yogurt
Monterey Jack cheese
Mayonnaise
Mozzarella cheese
Heavy whipping cream
Parmesan cheese
Sour cream
Swiss cheese

## Ketogenic Beef

- Corned beef
- Baby back ribs
- Prime rib
- Roast beef
- Steak
- Hamburger
- All cuts that are not lean

## Ketogenic Pork

- Ground pork
- Tenderloin
- Pork chips
- Pork roast
- Bacon
- Unglazed hams

## Ketogenic Poultry

Chicken broth
    Chicken eggs
    Cornish hens
    Whole chicken
    Chicken legs, wings, and thighs
    Canned chicken (read labels!)
    Turkey legs
    Ground turkey
    Whole turkey
    Turkey breast
    Pheasant eggs and meat
    Goose eggs and meat
    Duck eggs and meat
    Quail eggs and meat

## Ketogenic Seafood

Tuna fish
    Lobster
    Tilapia
    Flounder
    Shrimp
    Cod
    Scallops
    Canned salmon and tuna
    Salmon
    Anchovies
    Orange Roughy
    Haddock
    Herring
    Crab
    Trout

Catfish
Sole
Bass
Shellfish
Oysters
Sardines
Halibut

## Ketogenic Spices

Turmeric
Pepper
Pumpkin spice
Parsley
Paprika
Oregano
Onion powder
Hot sauce
Horseradish
Garlic salt
Garlic powder
Dill
Cumin
Cream of tartar
Cinnamon
Chili powder
Capers
Cajun spice
All spice
Real bacon bits
Salt

## Ketogenic Sauces and Dressings

Low-carb salsa
  Lime juice
  Lemon juice
  Italian
  Ranch
  Blue cheese
  Sugar-free syrup
  Sugar-free ketchup
  Yellow and brown mustards
  Worcestershire sauce
  Vinegar
  Soy sauce

## Ketogenic Liquids

Unsweetened tea
  Protein shakes
  Coffee with heavy cream
  Coconut milk
  Cashew milk
  Almond milk

## Ketogenic Sweeteners

Xylitol
  Stevia drops
  Erythritol

## Ketogenic Cooking and Baking

Cocoa powder
  Chia seed

Flax seeds
Flax meal
Almond flour and meal
Coconut flakes
Coconut flour
Sunflower oil
Sesame oil
Peanut oil
Olive oil
Mayonnaise
Hollandaise sauce
Duck fat
Coconut oil
Bacon fat
Butter
Béarnaise sauce

# 4

# Tips for Ketogenic Success

The main goal when you start the journey to better health via the ketogenic diet is to keep your body in a constant state of ketosis. For those that have personally utilized the diet, many have stated in excitement about how good they feel and look. This chapter is full of foolproof ways to keep yourself on track as you venture down the ketogenic road!

## *Hydration*

THIS SHOULD BE something you do daily already but consume 32 ounces of water within the first hour that you get out of bed in the morning and strive to drink up another 32-48 ounces before the noon hour. Drink ounces of water that is at *least* half of your weight or close to your full body weight in ounces daily to keep your overall hydration at healthy levels.

## Practice intermittent fasting

Start reducing your carb intake to a few days before getting down and dirty on the ketogenic diet. Break your day down into two phases:

- **Building phase:** Amount of time between first and last meal
- **Cleaning phase:** Amount of time between the last and first meal

START with a 12-16-hour cleaning phase and an 8 to 12-hour building phase. Your body will adapt over time, which will enable you to move to a 4-6-hour building time paired with an 18 to 20-hour cleaning phase each day. It will be much simpler to maintain levels of ketosis if you do this.

### *EAT tons of good salt*

WE ARE REMINDED ALL the time to lower our consumption of sodium. When you undergo a low-carb diet, insulin levels decrease, and our kidneys excrete higher levels of sodium. This results in a lowering of our sodium/potassium ratio.

- Add ¼ teaspoon of pink salt to glasses of water
- Add kelp, nori, or dulse to dishes
- Be generous with the amount of pink salt you add to food

- Consume pumpkin seeds or macadamia nuts as a snack
- Drink organic broth off and on throughout the day
- Eat cucumber or celery, both have natural sodium

## EXERCISE regularly

Daily high-intensity exercise help to assist in activating glucose molecules known as GLUT-4, which are responsible for reciting information to various areas of the body back to the liver and muscle tissues. This receptor takes away sugar that is in the bloodstream and uses it as muscle and liver glycogen. Exercising on a regular basis doubles the levels of crucial proteins in both the muscles and liver.

### Work on improving the mobility of bowels

If you are always constipated, ketosis will have a much harder time working its magic. Many people struggle with constipation issues while on the ketogenic diet. To help, consume fermented edibles, such as sauerkraut, coconut water, kimchi, etc.

It is recommended to take extra supplements, such as magnesium. Drinking one green drink per day will also help to increase the levels of calcium, magnesium, and potassium in your system, all of which help aid constipation and promote healthy bowel movement.

### Don't eat too much protein

Even though consumption of proteins is recommended by the ketogenic diet, some people do not know a proper balance and eat too much protein. Your body will change all those amino acids into glucose through the process known as gluconeogenesis if you eat too much protein. You will probably have to play with the amounts of protein you eat because some people need more or less than others.

### Choose your carbs wisely

The keto diet thrives on the elimination of carbs. But, it is best to consume at least some good types of carbohydrates, such as starchy veggies and fruits like berries, apples or citrus. Combine them into a green smoothie for a great morning pick-me-up!

### Use MCT oil

The usage of high-quality medium chain triglyceride (MCT) is crucial in keeping up with the state of ketosis. This is because this oil allows those that consume it to eat more carbs/proteins and still maintain a good level for ketosis. You can cook with this oil as well as add it into coffee, tea, green drinks, protein shakes, and more!

### Keep stress to a minimum

The build-up of daily stress will inhibit the process of ketosis. If you are under constant chronic stress, then now may not be the time to undergo the ketogenic diet, but rather a diet that concentrates on being anti-inflammatory and lower in carbs instead.

### Improve the quality of sleep

If you are not getting adequate amounts of rest, this is another aspect that can lead to a rise in stress hormones. Ensure that you are in a dark room that you feel comfortable in. It is recommended to get around 7-9 hours of sleep per night. The more stressed you are, the more sleep you need. Ensure that you are sleeping in a room that is no warmer than 65-70 degrees.

### Consume ghee

Ghee is a great substitute for butter, if not a total replacement! It is highly recommended while on the ketogenic diet and you can use it as normally as you utilize butter.

### Take Omega-3's

It is important to consume or take Omega-3 vitamins. Omega 3's should be more in your diet than Omega 6. Eating all that oil will cause you harm if your Omegas are not properly balanced.

### Avoid alcohol

While this sounds like a bummer, the consumption of alcohol can put a stop to your weight loss. Which is worth it: that bottle of beer or being able to fit into those clothes you are hanging on to in hopes you will once again fit into them?

### Make lemon water your best friend

Not only is it tasty and refreshing, but lemon water helps to balance out your pH levels, which can create the perfect environment for ketosis to properly thrive.

### *Avoid "sugar-free" products*

Even though it sounds better for you, try to avoid products that say "sugar-free" or "light" because these more than likely have more carbs than their original counterparts.

### *Avoid low-fat items*

While on the ketogenic diet, you should steer clear and not waste your precious time with anything that is low in fat. You need to have high percentages of fat in your diet to maintain an adequate and healthy balance. Otherwise, the protein you consume may be converted into sugars too.

### *Buy yourself a food scale*

This tool is important to have in your kitchen if you want total success on the keto. Being accurate is vital to the process of monitoring what you are fueling your body with. If you plan to track carbs and count calories, you really need to know what you are consuming. Make sure the scale you buy has a conversion button, an automatic shutoff, a tare function, as well as a removable plate.

### *Know healthy alternatives to carbs*

You will inevitably have cravings from time to time; no matter how successful you are while on the keto. There is something about fried chicken, rice, sauces, and more that make your mouth water. For ultimate satisfaction, it is a good idea to have alternatives and substitutes up your sleeve to combat cravings and not find yourself off the keto path. Try some of these alternatives!

- **Shirataki noodles** are low-carb and keto friendly, which makes them a perfect alternative when you have a hankering for pasta!
- **Cauliflower rice** can be used in the place of regular white or brown rice.
- **Spaghetti squash** can be creatively turned into noodles with the help of a spiralizer or simply with a fork. It has an awesome taste and less than half the carbs and calories.

- Use **heavy whipping cream** or **almond milk** in your coffee instead of that calorie-packed creamer.
- For those that love and constantly crave bread, there are many low-carb options, such as **low-carb breads and tortillas**!
- You will find that when your sweet tooth needs a bit of love that making shakes or smoothies with the help of **protein powder.** There are tons of flavors that can be easily mixed into batters, snacks, and much more! Plus, it gives you a nice boost of protein without sacrificing all the hard work you have put into the state of ketosis!

# 5

# Keto Breakfast Recipes

## Keto Egg Cups on the Go

*Ingredients:*

- 2 tbsp. cilantro
- Pepper and salt
- ¼ C. half and half
- 1 C. diced veggies, such as tomatoes, mushrooms bell peppers, onions
- 4 eggs
- ½ C. shredded sharp cheddar cheese
- ½ C. shredded cheese for the top

*DIRECTIONS:*

1. In a bowl, combine cilantro, pepper, salt, half & half, cheese, veggies, and eggs together.
2. Pour the mixture into 4 jars. Put on lids, but not too tight.
3. Pour 2 cups of water into your instant pot and then place a trivet over water.
4. Put egg jars on the trivet.
5. Cook on **HIGH** for 5 minutes.
6. Quickly release pressure.
7. Top the jars with ½ cup of cheese.
8. Broil for 2-3 minutes in an oven till the cheese melts and is lightly browned.

## Instant Pot Keto Breakfast Casserole

Ingredients:

- 1 ½ C. cooked breakfast sausage
- 2/3 C. peeled and grated sweet potato
- 8 eggs
- 1 C. chopped kale
- 2 tsp. minced garlic cloves
- 1 1/3 C. sliced leek
- 1 ½ C. water

DIRECTIONS:

1. Press the **SAUTE** button on your instant pot. Melt the coconut oil.

2. Add kale, garlic, and leeks to pot, sautéing till softened. Remove veggies and clean out the inner pot.
3. Combine sautéed veggies, sausage, sweet potato, and eggs in a bowl. Pour into a greased bowl or pan.
4. Pour water into the instant pot and place a trivet over the water. Add filled bowl carefully to pot onto the trivet.
5. Set to cook for 25 minutes on MANUAL. Perform a quick release of pressure.
6. Cut into slices and devour!

## Instant Pot Coconut Yogurt

Ingredients:

- 1 tbsp. gelatin
- 1 tbsp. raw honey or maple syrup
- 4 probiotic capsules
- 3 14-ounce cans of chilled coconut milk

DIRECTIONS:

1. With a spoon, take off solid cream off the top of cans of coconut milk and add to instant pot. Close and press the YOGURT. Adjust time till it says BOIL.
2. When the timer sounds, remove and let the bowl cool. With a thermometer, wait till it reads 100 degrees. This temperature allows cultures to grow.
3. Open the probiotic capsules and whisk into coconut cream.

4.  Place the bowl back into the instant pot and set the timer for 8 hours.
5.  Pour the mixture into a blender and add the gelatin gradually as you blend. Then, add additional flavoring of choice. (Honey, maple syrup, vanilla, etc.)
6.  Chill for a few hours to let cool and thicken. Enjoy!

## Instant Pot Hard Boiled Eggs

*Ingredients:*

- 1 C. water
- 16 eggs

## DIRECTIONS:

1.  Put a wire rack into your instant pot. Pour water over it.
2.  Put eggs on the rack.
3.  Press MANUAL to cook on HIGH for 4 minutes.
4.  When timer beeps, press CANCEL, and release pressure.
5.  Put into a bowl and pour in cool water. Let it sit for 5 minutes.
6.  Peel while warm and rinse off the remaining shell pieces.

## Overnight Apple Oatmeal

*Ingredients:*

- ¼ C. chopped pecans
- 1 C. chunky applesauce
- 1 ½ C. water
- ¼ tsp. pumpkin pie spice
- ¾ C. steel cut oats

*DIRECTIONS:*

1. Pour all ingredients into your crock pot. Stir well so it is combined well.
2. Cook for 8 hours covered and over low heat.

## Sausage and Egg Casserole

*Ingredients:*

- 8-ounces of shredded cheddar cheese
- 1-pound breakfast sausage
- 8 eggs

*DIRECTIONS:*

1. Grease your crock pot with cooking spray.
2. In a pan, fry the sausage.
3. Beat the eggs. Add half of the cheese and season with pepper and salt.
4. Pour the egg mixture into your crock pot and sprinkle

with cooked sausage. Top with the remaining cheese.
5. Cover and cook for 5 to 6 hours on low.

## Mixed Berry Cobbler Smoothie

*Ingredients:*

- 2-3 Medjool dates
- ½ C. blackberries
- ½ C. strawberries
- ½ C. blueberries
- ½ coconut milk

## DIRECTIONS:

1. Pour all ingredients into your blender.
2. Blend the mixture on high until you reach your desired texture.
3. Once smooth, add to a glass and enjoy!

## Butter Coffee

*Ingredients:*

- 1 tbsp. coconut oil
- 1 tbsp. grass fed butter
- 1 C. water
- 2 tbsp. coffee

## DIRECTIONS:

1. Brew coffee in any way you want.
2. Blend the coconut oil, butter, and brewed coffee in a blender for 10 seconds until light in color and creamy.
3. Serve and enjoy.

## Eggs Benedict

*Ingredients:*

- 1 tsp. chives
- 1 tbsp. white vinegar
- 4 slices of Canadian bacon
- 4 eggs
- 4 Oopsie rolls

## DIRECTIONS:

1. Separate 2 eggs and whisk together yolks until they double in volume. Add a bit of lemon juice.
2. Boil about 3 inches of water, reduce to simmer, add salt, and tbsp. of white vinegar.
3. With a wooden spoon, make a whirlpool in water by stirring a few times in one direction.
4. Crack an egg into a cup and lower into whirlpool gently. Don't drop the egg in, lower the cup and let it out.

5. Cook the egg for about 2-4 minutes, you want a runny consistency.
6. Lift the egg out with a spatula and let it rest on a plate lined in paper towels.
7. Repeat with the remaining eggs.
8. Fry the Canadian bacon however you like.
9. Top Oopsie rolls with bacon and place poached eggs on each slice of bacon.

## Blackberry Almond Chia Pudding

*Ingredients:*

- 2-3 tbsp. sliced almonds
- Drizzle of honey
- ¼ C. chia seeds
- 1 ½ C. vanilla almond milk
- 6-ounces fresh blackberries

*DIRECTIONS:*

1. Crush blackberries in a bowl with a fork until it is pureed.
2. Add honey, chia seeds, and milk to blackberry puree. Combine well and chill in the fridge overnight.
3. When serving, top with almonds and a few whole blackberries.

## Personalize Your Smoothie Bowl

*Ingredients:*

- 1 scoop of low-carb protein powder
- 1 tbsp. coconut oil
- 2 tbsp. heavy cream
- ½ c. almond milk
- 1 c. spinach

## OPTIONAL INGREDIENTS:

- 1 tsp. chia seeds
- 1 tbsp. shredded coconut
- 4 walnuts
- 4 raspberries

## DIRECTIONS:

1. Blend together the ice, cream, coconut oil, almond milk, and spinach until they are well-blended.
2. Pour in a serving dish.
3. Arrange toppings or throw them in and mix all together.

## Keto Morning Hot Pockets

*Ingredients:*

- ¾ C. mozzarella cheese
- 1/3 C. almond flour
- 2 eggs
- 2 tbsp. unsalted butter
- 3 slices cooked bacon

## DIRECTIONS:

1. Melt the mozzarella cheese and mix with the almond flour until combined.
2. Roll the dough out between a couple of pieces of parchment paper.
3. Ensure your oven is preheated to 400 degrees.
4. Scramble your eggs in the butter and place them within slices of bacon within the center of dough.
5. Fold over the dough to seal.
6. Bake for 20 minutes till golden in color and firm when touched.

## Keto Bagels

*Ingredients:*

- 1 tsp. baking powder
- 2 beaten eggs

- 3-ounces cream cheese
- 1 ½ C. almond flour
- 2 ½ C. shredded mozzarella cheese

## DIRECTIONS:

1. Mix the baking powder, almond flour, cream cheese, and mozzarella cheese together.
2. Melt in the microwave for 60 seconds, stirring well to combine.
3. Allow the mixture to cool a bit before adding eggs.
4. Divide the dough into 6 parts. With your hands, shape each portion into a round bagel.
5. Sprinkle each bagel with bagel seasoning mix or a pinch of sea salt if you so choose.
6. Ensure that the oven is preheated to 400 degrees. Bake bagels for 12 to 15 minutes until they start to turn gold at their edges.

## Breakfast Egg and Sausage Pie

*Ingredients:*

- 1 C. shredded cheese of choice
- 1 tsp. garlic salt
- 10 eggs
- 2 tbsp. coconut flour
- 1-pound of sausage

## DIRECTIONS:

1. Ensure your oven is preheated to 350 degrees.
2. Grease a deep-dish pie plate.
3. Mix the coconut flour and sausage together in the pie plate. Press the mixture along the bottom of the pie plate.
4. Crack your eggs into the plate over sausage. Sprinkle the eggs with garlic salt.
5. Bake for 45 minutes. Sprinkle with shredded cheese and then bake for another 15 minutes until the cheese has melted and eggs are totally set.

# Keto Lunch Recipes

**Juicy Instant Pot Chicken**

*INGREDIENTS:*

- 1 ½ C. organic chicken broth
- ½ tsp. salt
- ¼ tsp. pepper
- 1 tsp. dried thyme
- 1 tsp. paprika
- 2 tbsp. lemon juice
- 1 tbsp. coconut oil
- 4 pounds chicken
- 6 minced cloves garlic

*DIRECTIONS:*

1. Mix together the pepper, salt, thyme, and paprika. Rub the seasoning onto chicken.
2. Warm up the oil in your instant pot.
3. Place the chicken into the pot, breast side down, cooking for 6-7 minutes.
4. Flip over the chicken and pour in the broth, garlic cloves, and lemon juice.
5. Lock the lid and cook on **HIGH** for 25 minutes.
6. Allow the pressure to naturally release.
7. Remove the chicken and allow to cool for 5 minutes before attempting to cut.

## KETO MEATBALLS

*INGREDIENTS:*

- ¼ tsp. dried oregano
- 1 ½ pounds ground beef
- 1 tsp. dried onion flakes
- 1 tsp. salt
- 2 eggs
- 2 tbsp. chopped parsley
- 1/3 C. warm water
- ¾ C. grated parmesan cheese
- ½ C. almond flour
- ¼ tsp. pepper
- ¼ tsp. garlic powder

## TO COOK:

- 1 tsp. olive oil
- 3 C. keto marinara sauce

## DIRECTIONS:

1. Mix together all the meatball ingredients using your hands.
2. Form the mixture into 2" balls.
3. With olive oil, coat your instant pot.
4. Brown the meatballs in a skillet.
5. Layer the meatballs and marinara into your instant pot.
6. Set to MANUAL and push LOW to cook for 10 minutes.
7. Perform a quick release.
8. Serve with zoodles!

## CAULIFLOWER MASHED POTATOES

## INGREDIENTS:

- 1 C. water
- 1 head cauliflower
- Garlic powder
- Pepper and salt

DIRECTIONS:

1. Core the cauliflower and chop into chunks.
2. Place a trivet into the instant pot. Pour in the water and add the cauliflower to the trivet.
3. Close the lid.
4. Cook on MANUAL for 3-5 minutes.
5. Perform a quick release.
6. Take out the cauliflower and empty the inner pot.
7. With an immersion blender, puree till you reach the desired consistency.

## Broccoli Cheese Soup

INGREDIENTS:

- 1 tsp. pepper and salt
- ¼ tsp. garlic powder
- 1 bunch broccoli
- 1 C. heavy cream
- 1 C. shredded carrots
- 2 C. sharp cheddar cheese (shredded)
- 1 tbsp. onion powder
- 4 C. chicken stock

DIRECTIONS:

1. Turn the instant pot to SAUTE.

2. Place the butter in the pot and melt.
3. Pour in the pepper, salt, onion powder, garlic powder, chicken stock, carrots, and broccoli into the instant pot. Set to cook on HIGH for 5 minutes.
4. Perform a quick release.
5. Mix in the heavy cream and cheddar cheese.

## LOW-CARB CHIPOTLE FISH Tacos

*INGREDIENTS:*

- ½ diced yellow onion
- 1 chopped jalapeño pepper
- 1 pound of haddock fillets
- 2 pressed cloves of garlic
- 2 tbsp. Butter
- 2 tbsp. mayo
- 2 tbsp. olive oil
- 4 low-carb tortillas
- 4 ounces chipotle pepper in adobo sauce

*DIRECTIONS:*

1. Fry the diced onion with oil until translucent in color (for 5 minutes).
2. Lower the heat and add in the garlic and jalapeño and continue to cook, ensuring that you stir. Cook for another 2 minutes.
3. Chop the chipotles and pour them in with adobo sauce.

4. Add the fish fillets, mayo, and butter to the pan.
5. Mix everything together for around 8 minutes until the fish is cooked.
6. To make shells: fry the tortilla in a pan, frying for 2 minutes per side on high heat.
7. Let the shells cool and fill them with fish mixture.

# Keto Dinner Recipes

## Boneless Pork Chops

*INGREDIENTS:*

- Four to six pork chops (boneless)
- 1 C. water
- 1 package ranch mix
- 1 stick butter
- 1 tbsp. coconut oil

*DIRECTIONS:*

1. Put the pork chops in the instant pot along with the coconut oil.

2.  Push the SAUTE and brown all sides.
3.  Put the butter on top of the chops and sprinkle with the ranch mix.
4.  Pour water over pork chops.
5.  Put on the lid.
6.  Push the MANUAL and set to cook for 5 minutes.
7.  Allow the pressure to release naturally.
8.  Serve with buttery sauce over the top of the pork chops when serving.

## LOW-CARB GREEN CHILI Pork Taco Bowl

### INGREDIENTS:

- 1 tsp. pepper and salt
- 1 tbsp. olive oil
- 16-ounces of green chili salsa
- 2 pounds pork sirloin
- 2 tsp. garlic powder
- 2 tsp. cumin

### DIRECTIONS:

1.  Trim the pork and cut into slices against the grain.
2.  Mix the pepper, salt, garlic powder, and cumin together and then rub onto the pork.
3.  Press the SAUTE on the instant pot and brown the pork on all sides.
4.  Pour in the green chili salsa.

5. Lock the lid and push the MANUAL to cook on HIGH for 45 minutes.
6. Serve with the cauliflower rice.

## CRACK CHICKEN

*INGREDIENTS:*

- 1 C. water
- 1 packet ranch seasoning
- 2 pounds boneless chicken breast
- 3 tbsp. cornstarch
- 4 ounces cheddar cheese
- 6-8 slices of cooked bacon
- 8 ounces cream cheese

*DIRECTIONS:*

1. Put the chicken into the instant pot along with the cream cheese.
2. Sprinkle the ranch seasoning over the chicken and add water.
3. Set to MANUAL to cook on HIGH for 25 minutes.
4. Perform a quick release.
5. Take out the chicken and shred.
6. Set the instant pot to LOW and pour in the cornstarch.
7. Add the cheese and shredded chicken to the cornstarch.
8. Mix in the bacon and enjoy.

## JAMAICAN PORK ROAST

*INGREDIENTS:*

- ¼ C. Jamaican Jerk spice blend
- 4 pounds pork shoulder
- ½ C. beef stock
- 1 tbsp. olive oil

*DIRECTIONS:*

1. Rub down the roast with olive oil and spice blend.
2. Push the SAUTE on the instant pot. Brown the meat on all sides.
3. Pour in the beef broth.
4. Seal with the lid. Press the MANUAL to cook on HIGH for 45 minutes.
5. Perform a quick release. Shred pork and serve.

## SAUSAGE AND PEPPERS

*INGREDIENTS:*

- 1 tbsp. basil
- 1 can tomato sauce
- 1 C. water
- 1 can diced tomatoes

- 1 tbsp. Italian seasoning
- 10 Italian sausages
- 2 tsp. garlic powder
- 4 green bell peppers

## DIRECTIONS:

1. In your instant pot, mix the Italian seasoning, garlic powder, basil, water, tomato sauce, and tomatoes together.
2. Place the sausage in the instant pot.
3. Cut the peppers into long slices and pour the peppers on top of the sausage.
4. Lock the lid. Set the pot to cook for 25 minutes on HIGH.
5. Perform a quick release and enjoy!

# 8

# Keto Snack Recipes

**Green Bean Fries**

*INGREDIENTS:*

- ¼ tsp. black pepper
- ½ tsp. pink Himalayan salt
- 1 large egg
- 12 ounces of green beans
- 2/3 c. grated parmesan
- *½ tsp. garlic powder (optional)*
- *½ tsp. paprika (optional)*

*DIRECTIONS:*

1. Ensure that the oven is preheated to 400 degrees.
2. Ensure that your green beans are dry and ends are snipped.
3. On a plate, combine the seasonings with grated Parmesan cheese and mix together.
4. In a bowl, whisk an egg. Drench the green beans in the beaten egg and allow the excess egg to drop off the beans for a few seconds per handful.
5. Press the green beans in the parmesan cheese mixture and sprinkle cheese over them. Toss gently.
6. On a greased, large baking sheet, place the green beans evenly. Bake for around 10 minutes or until the beans are golden in terms of color.
7. Let the green beans cool so that you can consume with fingers. Serve alongside spicy mayo or ranch.

## Bacon-Wrapped Jalapeño Poppers

*INGREDIENTS:*

- 1 tsp. salt
- 1 tsp. paprika
- ¼ c. shredded cheddar cheese
- 16 fresh jalapenos
- 16 strips bacon
- 4 ounces of cream cheese

*DIRECTIONS:*

1. Ensure that your oven is preheated to 350 degrees.
2. Prepare 16 pieces of bacon cut lengthwise and in half.
3. Slice off ends of the jalapeños. Slice each pepper in half length-wise and ensure that you remove all the seeds and innards.
4. Mix the cheddar and cream cheese together.
5. Take the cheese mixture and proceed to fill each jalapeño half.
6. Engulf each jalapeño half with bacon.
7. Place the jalapeño poppers on a foil-lined baking sheet. Ensure that there is room between each popper. Bake for 20-25 minutes.
8. Add paprika, salt, and other spices to taste and enjoy.

## CRUNCHY KALE CHIPS

*INGREDIENTS:*

- 1 t. crushed red pepper
- 1 t. garlic powder
- 1 bunch of kale
- 1 t. salt
- 2 T. olive oil
- 2 T. Parmesan cheese

*DIRECTIONS:*

1. Ensure that the oven is preheated to 350 degrees.
2. Wash and thoroughly dry your bunch of kale.

3. Rip the kale into pieces, either leaving the stem on or cutting it off.
4. Pour the oil of choice over the kale and add seasoning.
5. Toss the kale and seasonings with hands to combine thoroughly. Almost every leaf should be shiny with oil.
6. On a cookie sheet, disperse the kale leaves evenly.
7. Bake the kale for 8 minutes. Check on them periodically. If the chips are still soft, continue to bake in 2-minute intervals. Average baking time is 12 minutes.
8. When crunchy to your liking, take them out and put in a bowl.

## CRISPY CHEDDAR CHEESE Chips

*INGREDIENTS:*

- 4 c. shredded cheddar cheese (or any blend you prefer)
- ½ tsp. sea salt
- ¼ tsp. chili powder
- ¼ tsp. cumin
- ¼ tsp. garlic powder
- ¼ tsp. paprika
- ½ tsp. onion powder

*DIRECTIONS:*

1. Ensure that the oven is preheated to 400 degrees.
2. With parchment paper, line a baking sheet, ensuring that

there is adequate room along the edges that will allow you to pick it up when hot.

3. Combine the cheese and spices in a bowl.
4. Spread out the cheese mixture evenly onto the baking sheet.
5. Bake until the cheese is visibly crunchy (about 20 minutes).
6. Take out of the oven.
7. Using parchment paper, lift out of the baking sheet.
8. Allow to cool for at least one minute and proceed to use a pizza cutter to cut cheese into triangles.

**Supreme Pizza Rolls**

INGREDIENTS:

- ¼ c. chopped green and red peppers
- ¼ c. pizza sauce
- ½ c. cooked and crumbled sausage
- 1 tsp. pizza seasoning
- 2 c. mozzarella cheese
- 2 sliced grape tomatoes
- 2 tbsp. chopped white onions

DIRECTIONS:

1. Ensure that your oven is preheated to 400 degrees.
2. With parchment paper, line a baking sheet, ensuring that

you leave extra room, especially along the sides so you are able to lift it out while hot.

3. Use a bit of olive oil to rub down parchment.
4. Sprinkle cheese on the baking sheet. It should be a single layer that covers the bottom.
5. Sprinkle the pizza seasoning over the cheese.
6. Stick in the oven and bake for 20 minutes up to the point that the cheese starts to turn brown in terms of color.
7. Remove from the oven and add the sliced tomatoes, red and green peppers, onions, and sausage. Then drizzle the tomato sauce all over the ingredients.
8. Bake for ten more minutes.
9. Take out of the oven and remove the pizza by lifting sides of the parchment paper.
10. Looking at your pizza horizontally, cut in 6 strips top to bottom. Then roll strips from top to bottom.

# Keto Dessert Recipes

**1 Carb Chocolate Glazed Meringues**

*INGREDIENTS:*

- 1 pinch of salt
- 1 ½ ounces of 90% cocoa dark chocolate
- 1 tsp. vanilla extract
- 1/16 t. liquid stevia
- 2 tbsp. unsweetened shredded coconut
- 4 large separated eggs

*DIRECTIONS:*

1. Ensure that the oven is preheated to 225 degrees.

2. Form soft peaks from the egg whites using an electric hand mixer.
3. Add a pinch of salt and sweetener and beat until stiff, white, and shiny peaks form.
4. Pour in the shredded coconut and vanilla extract. Fold these ingredients in gently.
5. Add meringue batter to a piping bag. You can use your own tip.
6. Cover a baking sheet with parchment paper and pipe the meringues into about 3" rounds.
7. Bake for 50-60 minutes.
8. Once baked, turn off oven and leave the door ajar. Let the meringues sit in the heat of the oven for 15-20 minutes to cool. This will prevent cracking.
9. Melt dark chocolate in a double broiler or in the microwave. Let chocolate cool for 10 minutes. Then pour on top of the meringues. (You can either drizzle chocolate over them or dip them into melted chocolate.)

**Caramel Nut Clusters**

*INGREDIENTS:*

BASE

- 1 tsp. coarse sea salt
- 20 macadamias
- 9 pecans
- 9 sugar-free caramel candies

Chocolate Ganache

- 2-3 tbsp. heavy cream
- ¼ tsp. vanilla extract
- 40 grams of 85% dark chocolate

## DIRECTIONS:

1. Ensure that the oven is preheated to 320 degrees.
2. With the parchment paper or foil, line a baking sheet.
3. Place the pecans evenly on a sheet and add macadamia nuts near them, making them overlap slightly.
4. Place a caramel candy onto each pile of nuts and put the sheet into the oven.
5. Bake for 10 minutes until the caramels are touching all the nuts. Do not allow the caramels to melt into large puddles.
6. While the caramels are cooling, heat heavy cream in a double broiler until it just starts to bubble. Drop the dark chocolate into the cream, and stir gently.
7. Once the chocolate is silky and smooth, add $1/2 - 1$ tsp onto each pile of nuts.
8. Sprinkle some sea salt on top while the chocolate is still wet.
9. Chill for about an hour and then feel free to enjoy!

## EASY KEY LIME Curd

## INGREDIENTS:

- One to two t. key lime zest
- 2 egg yolks
- 2 eggs
- 1 C. sugar substitute of choice
- 3 ounces unsalted room-temp butter
- 2/3 C. key lime juice, fresh

## DIRECTIONS:

1. In a food processor, process the sugar and butter together for 2 minutes.
2. Pour in the lime juice and combine.
3. Add the eggs one at a time, mixing for 1 minute once you have poured all of them in.
4. Process until the mixture appears curdled.
5. Pour into 1-cup mason jars and put on lids.
6. Pour 1 ½ cups of water into the instant pot and place the trivet over the water.
7. Put mason jars onto the trivet.
8. Lock the lid. Cook on HIGH for 10 minutes. Perform a 10-minutes natural release.
9. Take out the jars and open them carefully.
10. Sprinkle with lime zest and stir into the curd mixture.
11. Allow to cool with lids in for at least 20 minutes or overnight. It will thicken as it cools.

## ALMOND CARROT CAKE

. . .

## INGREDIENTS:

- ¼ C. coconut oil
- ½ C. heavy whipping cream
- 1 tsp. baking powder
- 1 C. shredded carrots
- 1 ½ tsp. apple pie spice
- ½ C. walnuts
- One C. almond flour
- 2/3 C. Swerve
- 3 eggs

## DIRECTIONS:

1. Grease the cake pan.
2. Combine all the recipe components with a hand mixer until it looks fluffy.
3. Pour into the pan and cover it with foil.
4. Pour 2 cups water into the instant pot and put a trivet over the water.
5. Place the cake pan onto the trivet.
6. Set to CAKE to cook for 40 minutes.
7. Allow to naturally release the pressure for 10 minutes and then release the pressure that remains.
8. Allow to cool before frosting it with your choice of frosting.

## BLUEBERRY LEMON CUSTARD Cake

. . .

*INGREDIENTS:*

- ½ C. coconut flour
- ½ C. fresh blueberries
- ½ C. sweetener of choice
- ½ tsp. salt
- 1 tsp. lemon stevia
- 1/3 C. lemon juice
- 2 C. light cream
- 2 tsp. lemon zest
- 6 separated eggs

*DIRECTIONS:*

1. Form soft peaks from the egg whites using a stand mixer. Set aside.
2. Whisk the yolks with the remaining ingredients minus the blueberries. Fold in the egg whites.
3. Grease the crockpot and pour in the batter. Sprinkle with blueberries.
4. Set to cook on low for 3 hours.
5. Allow to cook for at least 1 hour and then chill for at least 2 hours or overnight.
6. Serve ice cold with sugar-free whipped cream!

## Chapter 10: 21-Day Keto Meal Plan to Kick-Start Weight Loss

INSTEAD OF BASING your next New Year's Resolution around a diet that will do nothing but leave you stranded with disappointment and likely additional weight gain, this chapter will fulfill the doubts you have about making an adequate ketogenic diet meal plan.

Keep in mind that there is no one meal plan that fits everyone's body or overall lifestyle. You will likely need to make small adjustments to this meal plan, but it is a great starting point when you have no idea where to begin!

Contrary to popular belief, no, you do not need a ketogenic diet app on your mobile devices to be successful on the ketogenic diet with this meal plan.

### *Meal plan tips*

- Only cooking for one? Freeze or refrigerate any remaining servings or halve the recipes.
- Swap as you feel! This means you can eat lunch for dinner, breakfast for lunch, etc. You can even swap out entire days if you so choose. The sky is the limit.
- Whip up ketogenic buns in advance and freeze them to keep them fresh. Just make sure you defrost them the night before you plan to use.
- You will not need snacks or any meals in-between, but if you do experience hunger, make sure you have keto-friendly snacks on standby, such as:
- 1 hardboiled egg with pink Himalayan salt
- 2 to 3 celery sticks with 2 tbsp. almond butter
- Coffee with cream or almond milk
- Crispy bacon slices
- Fresh or frozen berries
- Ham and cheese roll-ups
- A handful of nuts and/or seeds
- Pork rinds
- Pour coconut oil into ice trays and keep in the fridge for a quick snack
- Diets that are extremely low in carbohydrates tend to be deficient in magnesium. It's recommended to take a

magnesium supplement or add snacks to your diet, such as nuts.

- If you do not feel hungry at regular meal time, drink water and don't eat if your body doesn't feel hungry.

- **Ketogenic Snack List**

WHEN I STARTED the Ketogenic Diet myself a couple of years back, one of the things I struggled with was edibles. I was able to quickly grab on the go that wouldn't throw my ketosis out of whack. That said, here is a list of snacks that are great to curb that appetite on the keto:

- 2 Celery sticks
- 1 cup Peeled Cucumber
- 2 tbsp. Almond Nut Butter
- 10 Kalamata Olives
- ½ Avocado
- 1 Boiled Egg
- Pecans
- Cashews
- Almonds
- Blackberries
- Strawberries
- Blueberries
- Walnuts Raspberries

# 21-Day Ketogenic Diet
# Meal Plan

For the recipes in this 3-week diet plan, simply click on the links to access them! The best part about this is that you can implement *any* of the recipes from the previous chapter into this meal plan to suit your needs and lifestyle.

You will find that the meals in this specific meal plan are very plain; the key to success when you start on any diet is simplicity and consistency. When you start to nail these two crucial things, then you can begin to incorporate other favorite recipes you enjoy making and devouring.

## Week One Recipes

**Chorizo Breakfast Bake**

*Ingredients:*

- 1 tbsp. olive oil
- ½ C. diced red pepper
- 2 large eggs
- ½ C. diced yellow onion
- 2 slices thick-cut bacon, cooked
- 4 oz. chorizo sausage

*Directions:*

1. Prepare the oven to 350°F. Two ramekins should be lightly oiled.

   2. Over medium stove settings, heat oil in a pan.

   3. Cook the onions and pepper on the pan until brown or for about 5 minutes.

   4. Fill the two ramekins with the vegetable mixture.

5. Add the chopped chorizo into the two ramekins.

6. Place the cracked egg into each ramekin then sprinkle with pepper and salt.

7. Place in the oven for twelve mins 'til the eggs are okay.

8. Top with crumbled bacon. Serve hot.

**Baked Eggs in Avocado**

*Ingredients:*

- 2 tbsp. cheddar cheese, shredded
- 1 medium avocado
- 2 large eggs
- 2 tbsp. lime juice

*Directions:*

1. Halve the avocado. Set the oven temperature to 450°F.

2. Take out some flesh from the middle part of the avocado.

3. Brush lime juice on the avocado halves and place upright on a dish.

4. Place cracked eggs on both avocado and sprinkle with pepper and salt.

5. Bake for ten mins. Add cheese to top.

6. Bake for additional three mins. until the cheese melts.

**Lemon Poppy Ricotta Pancakes**

*Ingredients:*

- ¼ C. almond flour
- ¼ C. powdered erythritol
- ¾ tsp. baking powder
- 1 large lemon, juiced and zested
- 1 tbsp. heavy cream
- 1 scoop egg white protein powder

- 1 tbsp. poppy seeds
- 10 to 12 drops liquid stevia
- 3 large eggs
- 6 oz. whole milk ricotta

*Directions:*

1. Mix ricotta, eggs, and stevia with half the lemon zest and the lemon juice within a food processor. Pour in a bowl after well-blended.

2. Mix in a pinch of salt, baking powder, poppy seeds, protein powder, and almond flour.

3. Over medium heat, heat a pan.

4. Pour ¼ cup batter into the pan.

5. Cook the pancakes, then flip.

6. Cook until brown and then place on a plate.

7. Cook the batter that is remaining.

8. Beat together the reserved lemon juice and zest, powdered erythritol, and heavy cream.

9. Drizzle the pancakes with lemon glaze and serve.

**Sweet Blueberry Coconut Porridge**

*Ingredients:*

- ¼ C. coconut milk
- ¼ C. coconut flour
- ¼ C. ground flaxseed
- ¼ C. shaved coconut
- ¼ tsp. ground nutmeg
- 1 C. unsweetened almond milk
- 1 tsp. cinnamon
- 60 grams fresh blueberries
- Pinch salt

*Directions:*

1. Over low heat, heat the coconut and almond milk in a saucepan.

2. Whisk in the salt, nutmeg, cinnamon, flaxseed, and coconut flour.

3. Raise the heat until the combination is bubbling.

4. Add in vanilla extract and the sweetener. Cook until it reached your desired consistency.

5. Place in two bowls. Put shaved coconut and blueberries on top.

**Sesame Pork Lettuce Wraps**

*Ingredients:*

- 6 oz. ground pork
- 4 leaves butter lettuce, separated
- 1 t. sesame oil
- 2 T. diced celery
- 2 T. soy sauce
- ¼ t. garlic powder
- 1 T. olive oil
- 1 T. toasted sesame seeds
- ¼ C. diced yellow onion
- ¼ C. diced green pepper
- ¼ tsp. onion powder

*Directions:*

1. Over medium stove setting, heat the oil in a pan.

2. Sauté the celery, peppers, and onions until tender. (5 minutes)

3. Add the pork to the mixture and prepare until brown.

4. Add the garlic and onion powder, sesame oil, and soy sauce.

5. Season with pepper and salt. Remove from heat.

6. Put the pork mixture on the lettuce leaves.

7. Serve with sesame seeds on top.

**Spiced Pumpkin Soup**

*Ingredients:*

- 1 small yellow onion, chopped
- ¼ cup heavy cream
- ¼ teaspoon ground nutmeg
- ½ cup pumpkin puree
- ½ teaspoon ground cinnamon
- one teaspoon minced ginger
- one cup chicken broth
- two cloves minced garlic
- 2 tablespoons unsalted butter
- 3 slices thick-cut bacon
- Salt and pepper to taste

*Directions:*

1. Let your butter melt over medium heat in a saucepan (large size).

2. Cook the ginger, garlic, and onions for up to four minutes. Ensure the onions are translucent.

3. Cook the spices next for another minute. Season with pepper and salt.

4. Boil together with the chicken broth and the pumpkin puree.

5. Remove from heat after simmering for twenty minutes on low heat.

6. Use an immersion blender to puree the soup. Simmer again for another 20 minutes.

7. In a separate pan, cook the bacon. Drain in paper towels.

8. Add the heavy cream and the fat of the bacon to the soup. Serve on top with the bacon that was crumbled.

**Easy Beef Curry**

*Ingredients:*

- 2 tablespoons curry powder
- 1-pound beef chuck, chopped
- 1 ¼ cups canned coconut milk
- one medium yellow onion, chopped
- one tablespoon grated ginger
- one tablespoon minced garlic
- one teaspoon salt
- half cup chopped cilantro, fresh

*Directions:*

1. Blend the ginger, garlic, as well as onion in a blender until it turns into a paste.

2. Cook the sauce for three minutes in a saucepan.

3. Add the coconut milk and for ten minutes, gently simmer.

4. Put in the salt, curry powder, and chopped beef.

5. Make sure to stir well before simmering for twenty minutes, covered.

6. Cook the beef thoroughly for another twenty minutes, simmering and uncovered.

7. Season to taste. Add freshly chopped cilantro as garnish.

**Rosemary Roasted Chicken and Veggies**

*Ingredients:*

- Salt and pepper
- 4 deboned chicken thighs
- 3 tablespoons olive oil
- 2 teaspoons fresh chopped rosemary
- 2 small carrots, peeled and sliced
- 2 cloves garlic, sliced
- 1 tablespoon balsamic vinegar

- 1 small parsnip, sliced and peeled
- 1 small zucchini, sliced

*Directions:*

1. Set the temperature of your oven to 350°F. Prepare a baking sheet (small rimmed) and grease lightly with cooking spray.

2. On a baking sheet, arrange the chicken thighs. Use pepper and salt to season.

3. Surround the chicken with veggies. Add sliced garlic on top.

4. Combine all the other ingredients by whisking. Then pour them above the vegetables and chicken.

5. Oven-bake for thirty minutes. Next, let it boil for about five minutes until the skin is crispy.

### Cheesy Sausage and Mushroom Skillet

*Ingredients:*

- ¼ cup marinara sauce
- ¼ cup water
- ¼ teaspoon dried thyme
- ½ cup shredded mozzarella cheese
- ½ teaspoon dried oregano
- 1 small yellow onion, chopped
- 1 tablespoon coconut oil
- 4 ounces sliced mushrooms
- 6 ounces Italian sausage, crumbled
- pepper and Salt

*Directions:*

1. Set the oven temperature to three hundred and fifty degrees Fahrenheit.

2. On a cast-iron pan and medium heat, heat oil until smoking.

3. Cook the sausages on the pan. Ensure it is brown and cooked through.

4. Let it cool in a cutting board for a while.

5. Cook the onion and mushroom in the same pan for about four minutes.

6. Add sliced sausages to the pan.

7. Add the pepper, salt, thyme, and oregano.

8. Add water and sauce. Stir them well. Oven-bake your pan for ten mins.

9. Add mozzarella on top. Cook until it melts (about five minutes.)

## Lamb Chops with Rosemary and Garlic

*Ingredients:*

- Salt and pepper
- 2 lamb chops, bone-in
- one t fresh chopped rosemary
- one T olive oil
- one T coconut oil, melted
- one T butter
- 1 clove garlic, minced
- ¼ pound fresh asparagus, trimmed

*Directions:*

1. In a shallow dish, add the garlic, rosemary, and coconut oil.

2. Marinate the lamb chops in the marinade overnight.

3. Set the marinated lamb chops aside for half an hour.

4. Over medium to high heat and a large pan, heat the butter.

5. Cook the marinade with the butter for six minutes. Use pepper and salt to season.

6. Flip the lamb chops on its other side for another six minutes.

7. Set aside the lamb chops for five minutes.

8. Season the asparagus with pepper, salt, and olive oil before placing on a baking sheet.

9. Char the asparagus in the broiler for eight minutes. Shake occasionally. Serve with the lamb chops.

### *Week TWO Meal Plan*

## Week Two Recipes

**Fat-Busting Vanilla Protein Smoothie**

*Ingredients:*

- ¼ cup vanilla almond milk
- ¼ cup whipped cream
- ½ cup heavy cream
- 1 scoop (20g) vanilla egg white protein powder
- ½ teaspoon vanilla extract
- 1 T coconut oil
- 1 T powdered erythritol
- 4 ice cubes

*Directions:*

1. Mix in a blender all the ingredients besides the whipped cream.
2. Blend until smooth.
3. Add whipped cream on top of the smoothie. Serve.

**Pepper Jack Sausage Egg Muffins**

*Ingredients:*

- ¼ teaspoon garlic powder
- ½ cup diced yellow onion
- ½ cup shredded pepper jack cheese
- 10 ounces ground breakfast sausage
- 2 tablespoons heavy cream
- 3 large eggs, whisked
- Salt and pepper

*Directions:*

1. Prepare three ramekins by spraying cooking spray. Make sure 350°F is the set temperature of your oven.

2. Mix together the pepper, salt, garlic powder, diced onion, and ground sausage.

3. Place the mixture in each ramekin.

4. Blend well the pepper, salt, heavy cream, and eggs.

5. Place the egg mixture in each sausage cup. Add shredded cheese on top.

6. Bake the ramekins for thirty minutes.

**Easy Cheeseburger Salad**

*Ingredients:*

- ¼ cup shredded cheddar cheese
- 1/3 cup diced tomatoes
- ½ teaspoon ketchup
- 1 teaspoon mustard
- 1 tablespoon diced pickles
- 3 ounces chopped romaine lettuce
- 3 tablespoons mayonnaise
- 7 ounces ground beef
- Pinch smoked paprika

- pepper and salt

*Directions:*

1. Cook the ground beef until brown over high heat. Use pepper and salt to season.

2. Remove the excess fat from the beef. Then, turn off the stove.

3. Blend the paprika, ketchup, mustard, pickles, and mayonnaise into a blender until smooth.

5. Mix the cheddar cheese, tomatoes, and lettuce in a different dish.

6. Coat the ground beef evenly with the dressing. Serve.

**Chicken Zoodle Alfredo**

*Ingredients:*

- ¼ cup grated parmesan cheese
- ¼ cup heavy cream
- 1 tablespoon olive oil
- 2 (6-ounce) chicken breasts
- 2 tablespoons butter
- 200 grams zucchini
- pepper and salt

*Directions:*

1. In a large skillet, warm the oil over medium-high stove setting.

2. Use pepper and salt to season the chicken.

3. Cook each side of the chicken in the skillet for 7 minutes.

4. Add the butter to the same pan over medium-low heat.

5. Place the parmesan cheese and heavy cream. Cook until it became thick.

6. Use spiralizer to cut the zucchini. Add them to the sauce mixture and chicken.

7. Let it cook for two minutes or until the zucchini is tender.
**Cabbage and Sausage Skillet**

*Ingredients:*

- ¼ cup mayonnaise
- ¼ cup sour cream
- ½ head green cabbage, sliced
- 2 tablespoons butter
- 6 large Italian sausage links
- pepper and Salt

*Directions:*

1. Cook the sausage in the pan. Slice them after.
2. Add the butter on the same hot skillet.
3. Add and cook the cabbage for four minutes until wilted.
4. Add the sliced sausage, mayonnaise, and sour cream into the cabbage.
5. Season with pepper and salt. Simmer for ten minutes.
**Gyro Salad with Avo-Tzatziki**

*Ingredients:*

- 6 cups chopped romaine lettuce
- 4 teaspoons lemon juice, divided
- 1 t fresh chopped dill
- 2 t fresh chopped mint
- ¼ cup chicken broth
- 1 medium ripe avocado
- 1 pound ground lamb meat
- 1 T olive oil
- ½ t dried thyme
- ½ teaspoon dried oregano

- ¹/₂ medium yellow onion, diced
- ¹/₂ English cucumber

*Directions:*

1. Over medium-high stove setting, warm the oil in a skillet.

2. For three minutes, add the lamb and stir occasionally. Add the onions.

3. Cook the lamb thoroughly. After the onions have softened, add the thyme, oregano, lemon juice (2 t), and chicken broth.

4. Taste with pepper and salt. Simmer for five minutes.

5. The grated cucumber should be wrung out of moisture using a clean towel.

6. Process the dill with a pinch of salt, mint, 2 teaspoons lemon juice, avocado, and grated cucumber until they have a nice texture.

7. Place the gyro meat on chopped lettuce. Add avo-tzatziki (spoonful).

## *Week THREE Meal Plan*

---

# Week Three Recipes

---

**Easy Cloud Buns**

*Ingredients:*

- 3 large eggs, separated
- 3 ounces cream cheese, chopped
- 1/8 teaspoon cream of tartar

*Directions:*

1. Line a parchment paper with a baking sheet. Set oven temperature to 300°F.

2. Whisk the egg whites until they are the consistency of foam. Whisk the cream of tartar on the egg whites until they are opaque and shiny.

3. Beat the egg yolks and cream cheese in a different bowl until they are combined thoroughly. Add them to the egg mixture.

4. Place ¼ cup circle of batter on the baking sheets about two inches apart.

5. Bake the bun until it is firm (about thirty minutes).

## Bacon Breakfast Bombs

*Ingredients:*

- ¼ cup cubed butter
- 2 large eggs
- 2 tablespoons mayonnaise
- 4 slices thick-cut bacon
- Salt and pepper

*Directions:*

1. Cook the bacon until crispy.

2. Set aside the bacon. Chop and place in a corner. Reserve the grease of the bacon for later use.

3. Boil salt and water in a saucepan.

4. The eggs should be placed on the saucepan to be boiled for ten mins. Transfer them next to a water bath (iced).

5. Peel the eggs once they are cool, and then coarsely chop them.

6. Add butter to the chopped eggs and mash them together. Add the pepper, salt, and mayonnaise.

7. Add the grease of the bacon into the mixture and stir. Cover the mixture and place in a fridge for half an hour.

8. Make six balls from the egg mixture before rolling them on the crushed bacon.

9. Serve them right away.

## Three-Cheese Pizza Frittata

*Ingredients:*

- ¼ cup grated parmesan cheese

- ¼ cup ricotta cheese
- ½ (10-ounce) bag frozen spinach, thawed
- ½ teaspoon dried Italian seasoning
- 1-ounce sliced pepperoni
- 2 ½ ounces shredded mozzarella cheese
- 2 tablespoons olive oil
- 6 large eggs
- Salt and pepper

*Directions:*

1. Three hundred seventy-five degrees should be the set temperature of your oven. Use cooking spray to grease a pie plate.

2. Use the microwave to defrost the spinach for four minutes. Wring out the water once done.

3. Whisk together the pepper, salt, Italian seasoning, olive oil, and eggs in a bowl.

4. Stir in the drained spinach, parmesan cheese, and ricotta cheese until well-combined.

5. Get the pie plate and have the mixture poured into it. Top the mixture with pepperoni and mozzarella.

6. Oven-bake for about thirty to forty mins so that the eggs are well-set and the cheese is lightly browned.

**Mozzarella Tuna Melt**

*Ingredients:*

- ¼ cup mayonnaise
- ½ cup diced yellow onion
- 1 green onion, sliced thin
- 1 tablespoon olive oil
- 2 ounces shredded mozzarella cheese
- 2 large eggs, whisked

- 8 ounces canned tuna
- Salt and pepper

*Directions:*

1. Use the medium heat setting of the stove to warm up the oil in a pan.

2. Cook the onions until they look translucent. (It takes five minutes.)

3. Place the drained tuna in the pan as well as the other ingredients.

4. Taste with pepper and salt, and for about two minutes, cook until the cheese has melted.

5. Place them in a serving dish with sliced green onion on top.

**Avocado Egg and Salami Sandwiches**

*Ingredients:*

- 1 medium tomato, sliced into 4 slices
- 1 small avocado, sliced thin
- 1 teaspoon butter
- 1-ounce fresh mozzarella, sliced thin
- 2 ounces sliced salami
- 4 Easy Cloud Buns
- 4 large eggs
- pepper and salt

*Directions:*

1. Make sure that the cloud buns are baked well with a golden brown color.

2. Use the stove's medium heat setting to melt the butter.

3. In the same pan, crack the eggs. Sprinkle with just enough pepper and salt.

4. One the eggs are cooked, lay them on every bun.

5. Top the buns with salami, avocado, mozzarella, and sliced tomato.

## Mushroom Soup with Fried Egg

*Ingredients:*

- 1 cup vegetable broth
- 1 large egg
- 1 teaspoon butter
- 1 teaspoon olive oil
- 100 grams cauliflower, riced
- 2 tablespoons shredded cheese
- 3 tablespoons heavy cream
- 4 white mushrooms, sliced thin

*Directions:*

1. Use the stove's medium heat setting to warm up the oil.

2. Place the mushroom in the pan and cook for about six minutes until tender.

3. Stir in the heavy cream, vegetable broth, and riced cauliflower.

4. After seasoning with pepper and salt, add in the cheese.

5. Let the soup simmer so that it will have the desired consistency. Remove from heat after simmering.

6. Let the egg fry in the butter. Serve on top of the soup.

## Cheesy Single-Serve Lasagna

*Ingredients:*

- Dried oregano
- 3 tablespoons low-carb marinara sauce
- 3 ounces shredded mozzarella

- 2 tablespoons ricotta cheese
- 1 small zucchini (60g), sliced very thin into rounds

*Directions:*

1. In a bowl safe to use in a microwave, place a spoonful of marinara sauce.

2. Place zucchini slices (1/3 only) on top of the sauce. Add ricotta (1 tablespoon each) to cover them.

3. Repeat the layering of sauce, zucchini, and ricotta.

4. Place the rest of the zucchini and 1 T of marinara on the topmost layer.

5. Have some mozzarella sprinkled on top before placing in the microwave for four minutes. Ensure the cheese melts perfectly.

6. Serve hot with drizzled dried oregano on top.

**Crispy Chipotle Chicken Thighs**

*Ingredients:*

- ¼ t garlic powder
- ¼ t ground coriander
- ¼ t onion powder
- ¼ t smoked paprika
- ½ t chipotle chili powder
- 1 tablespoon olive oil
- 12 ounces boneless chicken thighs
- pepper and Salt
- 3 cups fresh baby spinach

*Directions:*

1. In a small container, mix in smoked paprika, coriander, onion powder, garlic powder, and chipotle chili powder.

2. Flatten the chicken thighs. Season both sides with pepper and salt.

3. Divide the thighs in two. Use medium-high heat stove setting to warm up the oil.

4. Place the chicken thighs with its skin facing down on the pan. Drizzle the spice mixture over.

5. Let them cook for about eight mins. Flip so that the other side can be cooked for about five minutes.

6. When almost done, immediately add the spinach and let them wilt.

7. Make a layer of wilted spinach and place the crisp chicken thighs over it before serving.

### Pepperoni, Ham, and Cheddar Stromboli

*Ingredients:*

- ¼ cup almond flour
- 1 ¼ cups shredded mozzarella cheese
- 1 large egg, whisked
- 1 tablespoon melted butter
- 1 teaspoon dried Italian seasoning
- 2 ounces sliced pepperoni
- 3 tablespoons coconut flour
- 4 ounces sliced cheddar cheese
- 6 cups fresh salad greens
- 6 ounces sliced deli ham
- Salt and pepper

*Directions:*

1. Line a parchment paper on a baking sheet. Set 400°F as the oven's temperature.

2. Use a bowl safe for microwave-use to melt the mozzarella cheese until it can be smoothly stirred.

3. Mix dried Italian seasoning, coconut flour, and almond flour in a different container.

4. Add the melted cheese in the combination of flour. Season with pepper and salt.

5. Place an egg on the mixture and form a dough. Place in the parchment paper afterward.

6. Put another parchment paper on top. Make the dough oval.

7. Cut diagonal slits with a knife on the edges so that the middle is left untouched.

8. Make a layer of cheese and ham slices on the middle part of the dough before folding the strips above them.

9. Before baking for twenty minutes, brush butter on its top.

10. Serve the sliced Stromboli with a small salad.

**Spring Salad with Steak and Sweet Dressing**

*Ingredients:*

- 1 tablespoon butter
- 1-ounce toasted pine nuts
- 2 slices thick-cut bacon
- 2 tablespoons fresh raspberries
- 4 cups fresh spring greens
- 2 tablespoons white wine vinegar
- 2 tablespoons olive oil
- 7 ounces beef flank steak
- Liquid stevia, to taste

*Directions:*

1. After cooking until crispy over medium-high stove setting, finely chop the bacon.

2. Blend thoroughly the liquid stevia, raspberries, olive oil, and white wine vinegar in a blender.

4. In a large container, mix the crumbled bacon, roasted pine nuts, and the spring greens.

5. Pour in the dressing before dividing into two separate plates.

6. Use the medium-high heat setting of the stove to melt the butter. Add the steak.

7. Add pepper and salt. For four minutes, sear one side.

8. Flip and then cook for another five minutes.

9. Serve the steak with the salad.

# Conclusion

Thank you for making it through to the end of *Ketogenic Diet for Beginners*. I hope the contents of this book were able to provide you with adequate information to get you started on the right path to a healthier, better version of yourself!

I hope that what you have absorbed has provided you with just the right information for you to make the decision to create and build a body that you will be proud to show off! I hope that it gave you the tools you will need to achieve your health and/or weight loss goals.

The next step is to get off that couch, throw away that bag of potato chips and get to work! Even though you have just read some pretty great information that could lead you to create an entirely new you (on the outside, that is), that does not mean that something is going to happen without you following the guidelines of the ketogenic diet and really becoming motivated into helping yourself feel more alive. Isn't it about time you stopped the excuses and actually did something for yourself and your health?

# Conclusion

I wish you much luck as you conquer the delicious recipes shared with you within this book and that you will spread the amazing results you will find from the ketogenic with loved ones. You have nothing to lose!

Finally, if you found this book useful in any way, a review on Amazon is always appreciated!